Healing With Universal Energy

And Living A Balanced Life

Cindy Walker

CINDY WALKER

The information contained in this book is intended to be educational and not for diagnosis, prescription, or treatment of any health disorder whatsoever. This information should not replace consultation with a competent health professional. The content of this book is intended to be used as an adjunct to a rational and responsible healthcare program prescribed by a professional healthcare provider. The author is in no way liable for any misuse of the material.

DEDICATION

For those who find themselves living with health problems and stuck in the medical community, like I was, this book is for you! And for those who love us... may you find peace, love and guidance to help along the way.

I would also like to send some love out to all of my friends and family for the comfort, support and guidance you provide on my journey. We didn't have to pick each other in this lifetime and without you I wouldn't be the person I am today.

PROLOGUE

When people hear the words spiritual healing most think of religion. But my journey had nothing to do with religion.

I was 16 years old, living with my Aunt and enjoying life as a teenager. On April 2, 1990 life as I knew it was forever changed. I was babysitting a friend's baby, Steven, who was 6 months old and spending time with my sister Dawn. We were in my car and I was driving us toward Kalamazoo, MI on B Ave. I don't have detailed memories of the day or what happened. I just remember waking up in the intensive care unit at Borgess Hospital, being told that I was in a car accident and that my sister and baby Steven were both dead. I remember asking what had happened and having people question me for answers I didn't have. No amount of reading or study will prepare you for a tragedy of this magnitude. It felt like my entire world was in a vacuum and my "flight" response was triggered. I wanted out, wanted to be with my sister and remember telling the doctor to just let me die too. He said No.

Some people ask what it's like to die and come back. My experience wasn't like any of the stories you may have read about. I left my body and was forced back into it. There was no "light at the end of a tunnel." It was my soul, in pure energy form, reaching out and being pulled back in. It felt like a vortex of energy sucking me back into my body.

I had sustained major internal injuries and was hooked up to all these tubes and machines. I remember seeing a priest in my room who had offered to read the bible with me. My family wasn't religious and I had no idea what he was talking about so I sent him away. He came back to visit a few more times offering the bible during my hospital stay but I wasn't interested.

The doctors had to remove about 18 feet of intestine and decided to leave my abdominal cavity open to monitor and help with the gangrene infection that filled my core. My sternum was shattered and I had broken ribs along with a punctured lung. I'm not sure how long I was in the hospital but I remember Aunt Penny being there every day and watching the seasons change from the window. The day they sent me home was the day I watched them sew up my abdomen. No one knew the outcome for my life and I remember the Doctor telling my mom 6 months. I was sent home with a long list of instructions, an ileostomy, and colostomy, drain tube in my chest, IV and pain pump. I remember asking the doctor what I should do and he said with a smile "avoid stress." I didn't really know what stress was but I agreed to avoid it!

I lived in the medical community. Pills, surgeries and doctor visits had become my life. They were able to put my intestine back together eliminating the ileostomy and colostomy but the scar on my abdomen after surgery started growing out as it healed. I then needed plastic surgery and radiation treatment to stop the scar growth. Physically I was alive but emotionally I was a wreck. I weighed less than 100 pounds and had long, thin hair. Weak from all the health care. Leaving others to wonder how I was still alive. Through all this I never considered myself handicapped.

I believe eliminating that belief helped me more than if someone in my life would have encouraged the opposite.

Needless to say... when I realized 6 months had passed and I wasn't going to die, I became a rebel! I stopped listening to the doctors and stopped taking the medications. When I was 19 I met a man, got married and smoked a lot of weed! Because I chose to smoke marijuana I didn't spend much time in the medical community for fear they would discover my habit. Back then it was illegal to even possess this herb let alone use it for healing.

Several years passed, I was pain and health problem free. I lived a normal life, smoking weed, working and spending time with family. My husband believed marijuana could heal and was good for any ailment. I thought he was nuts but perhaps he was right. We eventually grew apart and divorced. I stopped smoking weed and went back to school. Along with completing courses to become an insurance agent I also studied hypnosis and became a Hypnotherapist.

The years passed and life progressed. I had chronic pain develop in my low back where I had sustained injury from the seatbelt. In 2006 I went to see a plastic surgeon and asked if there was anything he could do for my right hip/low back area. I had the remains of a hematoma from the seat belt injury and over the years it had become a place where fluid would build up. I was searching for relief with hopes of having it look better.

After meeting with the plastic surgeon and forming a plan, I decided to have the surgery. After surgery I was bruised all the way up my back and could only feel part of my right leg. Needless to say I wasn't happy with the results! When I met the doctor for my follow up appointment I learned he had performed liposuction on my right hip, back, butt cheek and thigh. Not the surgery we had agreed to. He said it looked great and I wondered if he was serious! Who has liposuction on only one side of their body! He had actually made it worse.

That was the end of my career as I knew it and the beginning of years of pain management, pills and searching for someone to help correct the mistake he had made.

In 2009 I moved to Arizona to go to the Mayo Clinic hoping they would have the cure I was looking for. Except they didn't have any new suggestions for treatment and I was stuck in the cycle of pain management, pills and physical therapy. After a couple of years the pain management doctor suggested a spinal cord implant. The long term goal was less pain medication and more mobility.

After another year and pressure to have the procedure I agreed to the trial implant. It did help and felt like I had an internal massager that activated the nerves to my right leg. So I went ahead with the permanent implant. Unfortunately the device was recalled. My long term goals were not met and I was left with additional pain, a brain tumor and full body Complex Regional Pain Syndrome (CRPS). My peripheral nervous system which involves nerve signaling from the brain and spinal cord which are all a part of the Central Nervous System had been damaged.

At that point I remember feeling like death would have been kinder. I had to literally beg doctors to see me and, if they did, I was begging to have the device removed. No one wanted to help me. I remember the last spine surgeon I spoke with telling me if I went to the brain surgeon and had the brain tumor taken care of he would consider removing the implant. It wasn't a yes, but it was all he had to offer. So I made an appointment with pain management to obtain a referral and went to see the brain surgeon.

After meeting with him, he wasn't concerned about the brain tumor and said my body would most likely absorb it over time. He asked if there was anything else he could do for me. I just started crying and asked him if he would remove the implant. At this point I thought he would say no like all the others, but he didn't. Instead he had a serious talk with me. His specialty was the brain, not the spine so if he were to remove the implant there was a high possibility that paralysis or death would result. I knew keeping the implant was the same risk so I accepted his help. After the removal surgery I felt better than I had in a long time and my 2 week follow up appointment the doctor was surprised with my recovery. He really thought I was going to be paralyzed from my chest down.

In the fall of 2013 I moved to Fairfield Iowa, a small meditation town in the middle of corn fields. I was still on a lot of medications and healing. A year before moving I had started to meditate regularly and changed my diet to incorporate more organic foods and less junk food. At this point in my life I didn't know what to do with myself. I had been trained on the pill diet and lived in the medical community for so long that my first goal after the move was to get myself back into that lifestyle. Well, the medical community here refused to see me as a patient! They were not equipped to care for someone like me. I was devastated! I didn't know what I was going to do so I began to meditate asking for clarity and guidance.

What I received... I had 2 choices... I could relocate again to continue on with life in the medical community. Or I could stay in Fairfield, step myself off the pills and find a different way of living.

Sometimes our emotions get in the way of making logical choices. I was really upset and felt as if I been kicked out of the medical community that I grew up in. When I took a step back and examined the 2 options I had before me there was only one logical choice. What I had been doing for most of my life, living in the medical community, wasn't working. The combination of horrendous side effects from all of the pills, getting worse physically, and the mental stress was really taking a toll on me. I had moved to this little town in Iowa seeking peace and a better, healthier way to live. I didn't think it was fair for me to give up because I felt the need to refill the pill bottle. I was lead to this little town for a reason... at the time of this writing 2 years have passed since

I took the second option. Against the advice of every doctor I have ever spoken with, I decided to take my life back, minus one pill at a time. It was the best decision I have ever made. Not as hard as the medical community makes it out to be.

I wish I would have taken this option sooner.

When you are living inside of the medical community you find yourself searching for others to help you heal. You think perhaps there is a pill or a surgery that will cure you. I lived like that for most of my life; I was continually searching outside of myself for the latest and greatest "cure." What I learned along the way was that the "cure" I was looking for was already inside of me. I just needed to change my focus. You would think that someone with my training in hypnosis would already know this! And I did, for others. I was helping others and searching for someone to help me. Seems silly to admit yet I know most of the world is programmed like this.

At one point in my journey I had given up on myself because someone I loved said "if you can't help yourself, how can you help others?" This person was an abusive narcissist and it seemed no matter what I did, nothing was ever right and I couldn't help them. So, pain medication in hand, I fell into the self-destructive emotional spiral they offered me. It wasn't until I was able to get this person out of my life that I was able to move forward.

December 2013. I had a plan. I counted all the pills I had left and researched the proper way to decrease the dose of each medication. I felt that if I were to go "cold turkey" and stop every medication at the same time that I would experience severe withdraw. I live alone and wasn't welcome in the medical community here. Failing was not an option! So I made a 2 week plan with the end result to be drug free. I ordered some herbs, kava and CBD oil, to help with withdraw symptoms I expected to have. I was determined and prepared.

After a couple of days I noticed very few withdraw symptoms and found that what I did have I could control with meditation, calming my mind and having an internal conversation with my body and they went away. At the end of the first week I was off all the medications and my mind felt awesome! It was like tasting freedom for the first time! I was diffusing essential oils in the house, meditating and ready to start a new chapter of life. I didn't even need the herbs and still have them in the cupboard as a reminder.

To those reading this and wondering if you should stop taking your medications. I suggest you speak with your health care provider before doing this, look at all your options and make a logical decision that's best for you. I was taking morphine, lyrica and using a 7 blend narcotic body lotion to sustain the conditions I had.

Am I healed? I'm not sure I will ever be 100% healed. But I am positive and grateful for the a new chapter of life. I'm missing organs and have scars left behind as a reminder of the journey. I still have pain from time to time and occasionally my blood will pool in my feet.

I don't keep track of the bad days anymore. I meditate, do my best to make healthy food choices, adding more minerals & herbs into my diet, I'm spending more time in nature and look forward to the positive side of my life journey. Once I changed my focus from sustaining what I had to actual healing the past and growing into the future, things changed for me. Our purpose in life is to create an atmosphere. I've learned to be mindful of the atmosphere I am creating for myself and the experience others have inside it.

The choices I made on my journey are just that, my choices. Looking back I have no regrets. The lessons I learned along the way are priceless. Without them I wouldn't be here today helping others.

A few things I noticed about the medical community

- o They don't talk about the body's natural energy, the chakra system and the role it has in the composition of the human body.

- o Their main focus is the physical body omitting treatment of the spiritual/soul nature of the person.

- o It's very rare you will find a physician in the medical community suggesting what is considered alternative medicine or therapy.

Once I realized this gap in treatment I started searching for alternative therapies and Spiritual Healers. I knew I needed more, even though I wasn't sure what that "more" consisted of. While researching Healers I discovered that I was able to work with entities from the spiritual realm for my personal healing and also able to offer their services to others. Think about it like this.. if Granny was a brilliant Doctor in the physical world and has changed back to pure energy in spiritual form she didn't forget the lessons she learned in life. She still has the ability to use her skills and help others who are physical. The only difference is, she is now considered an entity in spiritual form.

As a young child I used to have nightmares of the world, see spirits and knew things about others that I couldn't explain. Back then it was taboo to talk about those things and if I did I was treated like an outcast. Because of this it took me several years to accept the psychic medium side of myself. When I started meditating on a regular basis for healing and working with the entities more of my abilities started developing.

I can see and/or hear the entities so why not ask them for advice. This gift comes in handy when helping others or seeking guidance for myself. Not sure why I was so scared of this ability growing up. Perhaps it was because of the way others reacted around me. If you find yourself in this position, with abilities, the best advice I can offer is to follow your instincts, meditate and ask the spiritual realm for guidance. As physical beings we spend so much time functioning in an imperfect physical world that we forget we are pure energy and where we came from.

TABLE OF CONTENTS

The following information is divided into two sections for those who are seeking spiritual healing and guidance through meditation, along with a greater understanding of the chakra system.

Section 1 ~ Page 1
Meditating and asking for Spiritual Healing

- o How to summon Angels, Entities, Spirit Guides and other non-physical friends and family

- o What can you expect?

- o What does healing look like?

- o Clearing spiritual attachments

- o How to prepare for meditation with spiritual Healing

- o How to meditate

- o Channeling the energy

- o Trusting the non-physical messages you receive

Section 2 ~ Page 15
A Basic Understanding of Your Chakras and Aura

- o The concept of Universal Energy

- o A brief explanation of the Law of Attraction

- o What are Chakras and Aura

- o 7 Chakras Explained

- o How Chakras radiate energy into the Aura

- o 7 layers of Aura Explained

- o The Power of Colors

- o Can you read Aura? With how to tips!

- o Balancing your energy for physical and emotional health

CINDY WALKER

SECTION 1 ~ MEDITATING AND ASKING FOR SPIRITUAL HEALING

When we are sick we are trained to ask others for help. So when asking for, and opening yourself up to spiritual healing it requires a different way of thinking. You are taking a leap of faith where what you commit to is to show up for yourself. Fully. Completely. All of you. With hope and trust that you'll be caught, held, and healed by something or someone larger than yourself. Reality is, your physical body is part of Nature, *you* are the one doing the healing and the entities are only there to assist you.

How to summon Angels, Entities, Spirit Guides and other non-physical friends and family

When someone leaves the physical body they reemerge into the wholeness that they really are. They go completely into the universal energy that is all around us. You have always had access to them within this energy whether they were physical or not. The only difference is when someone is physical we would pick up the phone or go to their home to speak with them. When they are no longer physical and we want to spend time with them our strong desire, thoughts and intentions serve as the connection.

People are really confused about non-physical. It's something that you like to think about sometimes but don't want to think about most of the time and because you don't understand it, and because there are so many really crazy stories that people tell about it, it becomes hard for us to remember who we really are. We are multi-dimensional beings. When we cross over to the non-physical we still have interest in all that we created while physical. So in the spirit of keeping this simple, focus, intention and desire. That is how you call upon spiritual entities. You do not need to call them by name as long as you verify your intention and understand that you have this unseen but not unknown, unseen but not unfelt, force of nature that is flowing with you.

You have access to as much as you are willing to ask for and you get to experience as much as you are consciously able to allow.

What can I expect?

Asking "Can I expect a miracle?" Feels like you are asking for a lot doesn't it, but the answer is Yes! I have always found it easier to ask with a specific outcome in mind with no expectations of how the outcome will be received.

Now, having said that, your miracle may not look exactly like what you'd expect.

Some things to keep in mind:

1. *Healing is a process, not an event.*

2. *You don't get what you want, you get what you need!*

You may need to heal another area or areas of your life first, *before* the specific area you had in mind. A physical illness may be connected to an emotional trauma or vice versa.

3. *Your healing may be instantaneous or rapid.*

   More often, though, it's a series of shifts and transformations. The Entities often assist in layers, each layer transforming as necessary and as you're ready. People who don't receive instant physical healing often have shifts in other areas of their life. Your challenge could well be an opportunity to grow.

4. *What you are dealing with right now might be something you have come into this life to experience.*

    It may be a soul contract or lesson you set up. And your soul's goal, no matter how difficult, and challenging is not to eradicate the challenge but to learn, grow and evolve because of and through it.

5. *Your whole being receives healing, something that you cannot direct or have control over.*

   Healing is not compartmentalized to certain aspects of yourself. You may think you have only physical issues or are only participating for your emotional health, but everything is connected and all of you will receive healing.

6. *Very occasionally, based on your soul contract, the Entities may say that they cannot help you.*

   If it is your lesson to experience something, they cannot change things or intervene. If this is the case, they will let you know.

*We are not human beings having a spiritual experience;
we are spiritual beings having a human experience.*

We are magnificent beings of Love, Wisdom, Beauty,
Truth, Power, Light, and much more. We incarnate as
human beings to experience life so we can evolve as souls.

Meditation helps you connect more deeply with your
spiritual nature and Higher Self. It also helps you connect
with the Divine, God, Goddess, Source, Spirit, or whichever
term you use for the Sacred and Transcendent. When you
open up to who you are as a soul you allow the Transcendent,
Grace, Love, and Light to enter you. This alone can clear and
heal many layers.

Healing begins once you decide to participate and
intensifies during the session. Each moment is a wonderful
opportunity to be with, process, shift, and let go of those
things that are no longer serving you. Allowing you to heal
and evolve. You may think you receive healing only while in
meditation, but if you tune in to your higher self, in silence
and reflection, you will discover that there is a lot more going
on.

A lot of the work is done at night, while you are sleeping,
when your resistance and defenses are down. You may have
vivid or significant dreams, some of which you understand
and some that will make sense later. Keep a note pad by your
bed and make note of them. You might find yourself awake
in the early hours of the morning, refreshed even after only a
few hours of sleep. Or that it's hard to sleep deeply.

*Every moment is a learning, growing, and healing
opportunity. There are teams of Entities assisting you. So
much incredible guidance and transformation is at hand,
just for you. Take advantage of it.*

What does healing look like?

Healing is holographic. This means that when the Entities are assisting you they are seeing you as a pure energy hologram, as a whole being with several interconnected aspects or layers: spiritual, emotional, physical, mental, energetic, karmic, soul purpose and past lives. They know every aspect of you and your life, including relationships, family, work, gifts and talents, financial, creativity etc., and want to help you heal and evolve.

The Entities also know all about your soul's journey, purpose and contracts. They assist your soul in its highest purpose. You came into this life with certain contracts and to learn certain lessons through various situations and relationships. They help you with every part of it. They help you to become aligned. Harmonious and connected to all that you are.

Sometimes people want only physical healing or spiritual growth. But holographic healing is about the whole. If you only want physical healing, it's likely connected to something that's not about your physical body, but about your emotional state, approach to life, relationships, or past life experiences. It could be that you need to learn or shift something outside of your illness. Likewise, if you focus only on your spirituality and ignore your sick body, the Entities will begin with the physical. Wholeness is including and integrating all aspects of your being, including the non-physical.

The Entities healing assistance is of a different paradigm than what you may be familiar with. They heal and assist through exalted vibrations of Light and Love.

Clearing Spiritual Attachments

Almost everyone has attachments, spirits who have attached themselves to us. The Entities are the best clearers of unwanted attachments.

Physical or mental illness is often attributed to a being or beings connected to a person. These beings could be a soul in limbo, a relative who has passed, a spirit randomly picked up, or a negative entity. These beings for whatever reason are not connected to the Light. Usually we have a corresponding vibrational "hook", like an emotion or belief, which attracts and links them to us.

The Entities, when asked, clear these attachments from us and transport them to the Light.

Healing is a series of levels, a series of shifts.

Each time you meditate and connect to your Higher Self, you're a little more ready to release what is no longer serving you. You've grown a little more. You're a little further along on your journey.

The Entities assist you where you are each time. Very gently, effectively, with incredible compassion, and understanding. They know things take time to be done; knots to be untied, relationships to be worked out and worked through. All of this takes time.

A lot of your healing is your own personal growth and this simply cannot be rushed. The Entities definitely help you with it. But this isn't something they can do for you. It's your responsibility.

Before meditation set time aside to emotionally and spiritually prepare. If any of the following questions resonate with you, take time to sit, reflect upon and answer them.

Why am I doing this?

What is this journey about for me?

What do I truly want to change?

Who would I be if I changed?

How would I feel if I changed?

What will the change mean for me?

Is this change within myself or outside of myself?

Is the reason I am doing this responsible for making me unhappy or stressed? or is there a deeper reason that I don't know about, that I may be afraid to face or cannot feel yet?

As you review your life, what do you want healing on?

What part of your life or yourself do you want to grow and transform?

Make a list of all the areas of your life. The following are some areas to get you started. You may even notice a few more:

Physical
Emotional
Energetic and psychic
Spiritual
Relationships
Work, career, life purpose
Money and material resources

Be open to all your experiences, thoughts, dreams, emotions, sensations, intuition, and energy. Stay open to your judgments, doubts, criticism, skepticism, negative emotions and resistance. Stay open to receiving in every obvious and subtle ways. Notice the shifts in perspective and aha moments. Stay open to images, messages, knowing's and guidance you receive. There are teachings and lessons everywhere and in everything.

Set aside time each day to reflect and meditate. The Entities begin ASSISTING you the moment you decide to participate, so you may feel their presence or an increase in energy AS SOON AS YOU focus on the request.

How to prepare for meditation with spiritual healing

Find a quiet place to relax and meditate, with no distractions, remind yourself of 3 things you would like to work on. This is how you invite the Entities to work on you. They won't barge in, they wait for an invitation!

Even though the Entities know everything about you, creating the requests you would like to focus on during the session are your participation in your healing process.

Place a glass/bottle of water beside you before you start meditation so the entities may bless and infuse it with energy. After meditation drink the water. You may also listen to guided meditation recordings or relaxing music during the session.

Although there are no specific rules to prepare for spiritual healing, you should be careful not to eat too much before mediation, or do anything straining or be socializing too much immediately after. This is probably a good time to be introspective and review in your mind the things that you asked for help with. Take note of any feelings and images that come to you in relation to your issue. Remove your watch or anything tight around your waist. Try not to have any straps across your heart either. Some find wearing white clothing helps but it's not required.

Some people feel the entities working on them and others do not. The fact that you felt nothing and you now feel energized does not mean you do not have major changes inside your body. You may feel euphoric because of the spiritual energy, but you should be very careful to notice the areas of your body that experienced healing and treat yourself with extra care.

Some people have asked why they started crying during session for "no reason." Should you find yourself in this type of release, it's okay. Emotions will come up. They may be deep and intense. They may be overwhelming or subtle, fleeting or lasting, dark or light. They are essential for your healing. The tears are a form of release. Let them flow.

When you feel difficult feelings like grief, pain, hurt, loss, disappointment, anger, hate and jealousy simply be with them. You don't have to do anything, often you cant. Just open to each emotional fully. When you do they will be lifted out of you.

What you need to learn is often outside of what you currently know. The path to learning and healing is through your feelings. This process leads you there. The Entities lead you there. All you need to do is participate by feeling and staying open to those things you do not know yet.

Keep your thoughts positive.

Let go of the idea of specific results, what "should occur" and when. Your healing might take a much different path than you think.

Pay attention to your intuition, synchronicities, etc.

Watch and Listen for what you don't know yet.

When you think you know, or have a specific belief on a subject, you create a lid or blockage limiting yourself and your world. When you stay open minded to what you don't yet know you are receptive.

Physical illness, even the most severe diagnosis, is an opportunity to heal or shift from within. It could be emotional healing by opening to love or living from joy and creativity or it could be spiritual healing by reconnecting in a new way with the Divine and your divinity.

Now that you know what to expect, and have your goals & intentions ready, the next step is to meditate. Meditation is very easy and you may even notice you are already doing some form of meditation in your daily life.

HOW TO MEDITATE

The goal of meditation is to focus and quiet your mind, eventually reaching a higher level of awareness and inner calm. You can meditate anywhere and at any time, allowing yourself to access a sense of tranquility and peace no matter what's going on around you. For those new to meditation you will enjoy the following suggestions to get the most out of your session.

Meditation should be practiced somewhere calming and peaceful with no distractions. This will enable you to focus on the goals and intentions you have set for yourself. Try to find a place where you will not be interrupted for the duration of your meditation - whether it lasts five minutes or half an hour. Some people like to meditate while in bed either right before they get up in the morning or before they fall asleep at night. When working with the entities I suggest meditation at bedtime so they are able to work on you while you sleep. But it's totally up to you when, where and for how long you meditate.

For those new to meditation, it's especially important to avoid any external distractions. Turn off TV sets, the phone or other noisy appliances. If you play music, choose calm, repetitive and gentle tunes, so as not to break your concentration.

Wear comfortable clothes and take off your shoes. One of the goals of meditation is to calm the mind and block out external factors. This can be difficult if you feel physically uncomfortable due to tight or restrictive clothing. Some people like to meditate in a sitting position and others like to lay down. As long as you are in a comfortable position the choice is yours.

Some people enjoy writing, drawing, painting, crocheting, pottery or other forms of creative relaxation that allows them to clear their mind and focus. There are many ways you can connect to the non-physical side of yourself. It's your choice. Do what makes you happy and is most comfortable for you.

When I was a young child I remember visiting my Grandmother and finding her lying on the floor in the living room. She picked the spot in front of the sliding glass door where the sun was shining in. I thought it was strange to see her on the floor and asked what she was doing. Her reply "I'm resting!" Had I known back then the things I know today I would have joined her! Part of me wishes she would have taken the time to explain and taught me how to find what my little soul needed.

Channeling the Energy

There are many different ways to view this subject. If you understand that we are both physical and non-physical then you understand that what some call channeling is really someone who is connected to the non-physical side and sharing information, translated through them, to others. The non-physical side of consists of pure universal energy, all that is or will ever be. Some consider this more than one Entity because different "things" have a different feeling within the energy flow. The non-physical is not separate like the physical is. Imagine it as a bowl of multi colored ice cream, when it's frozen it appears solid and separate but when it melts it combines and becomes one. It will still have all the different flavors but the look has turned into one flowing liquid.

When a Medium incorporates an Entity that Medium is allowing a specific flow of energy into their body. When you are inside this flow of universal energy you have access to infinite knowledge. Nothing is separate and we all have the ability to channel this energy.

When you learn to balance your energy between the physical and non-physical (meditation is the easiest way to begin) you will notice more of what you focus on showing up in your perceived reality.

Trusting the non-physical messages you receive

You know the difference between just feeling something and feeling something that resonates with source. Trust yourself and your intuition. You come from non-physical, and non-physical still remains non-physical, so you always have that relationship with non-physical, it's part of you and never goes away. This non-physical side of you is what your emotions are. So when you have an impulse to do something, if you are keenly aware of the way it feels, you can feel if you are resonating with source energy or not.

Your thoughts and emotions are what is creating the atmosphere around you and others. This atmosphere is where your messages are coming from. Be mindful of the atmosphere you are creating.

CINDY WALKER

SECTION 2 ~ A BASIC UNDERSTANDING OF YOUR CHAKRAS AND AURA

This chapter is filled with information to give you a basic understanding of our internal energy system. It breaks down aura color and why it is important to be able to see auras. I have included tips and methods to clean your aura that are practical and simple to apply. You will get an understanding of how to sense, cleanse, and balance your internal energy starting today so that you can start attracting the things that you have always needed and desired.

THE CONCEPT OF UNIVERSAL ENERGY

Everything in the universe is connected: people, events, nature, even places. We are all created out of energy that we pass along. The world and people around us are pulsating with an internal and external energy that we can pick up. We are miniscule drops of water in a vast ocean of universal energy. Some call this energy the universal mind. Have you ever wondered why no matter how hard you try you cannot achieve your goals? Nothing seems to go right for you? You cannot maintain the relationships you would like? Well my friends, it may be your own fault. Sorry to say, but your own negative energy may be the only thing standing in your way. Your own negative thought processes may be repelling what you want. No, it's probably not bad luck; it may be as simple as fixing your internal flow of energy. It may be as easy as cleansing your aura and freshening up your thoughts.

A brief explanation of what is called the law of attraction:

Everything and everyone in the universe is made up of energy.

Ideas and thoughts leave an energy trail.

What you think about, focus on, and put your energy into, you acquire; sometimes in excess.

Your emotions and feelings are energy that works like a magnet, the universal energy matches this energy by sending equal, echoing energy.

Now, you may already have conquered positive thinking. You may be doing all of the right exercises, using positive affirmations, visualizing the right things, and find you are still not getting what it is that you want.

Well, we have to remember a few things.

1. Our conscious brain is not always in tune with our spiritual mind. The two forms of energy must be in line and in agreement. Sometimes the spiritual mind knows better than our conscious mind.

2. Sometimes our spiritual and conscious mind are on

a different time schedule than the universe. It is all about timing.

3.   Our own internal energy flow has to be functioning at its best. It has to be free flowing and clean.

This is the one thing we have control over entirely. This is where the answer to our "problems" usually lies. We have the ability to cleanse our aura and allow our energy to flow freely throughout our spiritual body. Bad energy needs to be pushed out and blockages must be cleared. Some of those negative things are internal and some are external. Either way, you have the ability to fix it.

Our system is pumping and vibrating with universal energy. It flows through our chakras and out into our auras. Emotions and ideas change our energy flow and the type of energy that we have: be it positive or negative. When we clear blockages in our internal energy system and cleanse our auras, we will have positive ideas and exude positive energy. Guess what that attracts? You guessed it... positive things, events, and people.

The one thing that we can control is the type of energy we put off and the atmosphere you create around you. You can have control over your life, relationships, and circumstances.

The balance of our energy system directly relates to how well we are able to use the law of attraction to our advantage. All we need to do is balance our internal energy. The key to doing this is to learn about auras and chakras, how to clear them and how to cleanse our energy. This is how we become the captain of our ship instead of the prisoner.

WHAT ARE CHAKRAS AND AURA?

Our world is alive with energy, quite literally. Everything in us and around us gives off energy of some sort . The atoms in our cells are configured so that each has both negative and positive charges, our own tiny batteries. Our physical bodies are constantly emitting and taking in energy. This energy is our life force. It effects our bodily functions, our emotions, and our spirituality. In turn, it is also affected by all of these things.

Chakras and auras are both ways that we can view, channel, access, and interact with this life energy. The power plants, or hubs, for our life energy are our chakras. These spinning wheels of light and energy are usually characterized as a row of colored circles that run from the head to the genitals. Chakras , in reality, are actually spinning vortexes of color and light that radiate from the center of the body, both through the front and the back.

There are seven main chakras.

Each channels the flow of energy through our beings. Chakras are the regulators and gate keepers of our life force. The level at which our chakras function is a reflection of how we choose to handle circumstances in life. Our thoughts, feelings, and how we generally view the world around us determine how open or closed our chakras are.

Chakras are an extension of our awareness.

They have more mass than auras, but less than the body. Even though they are part of our consciousness, chakras play a part in the physical processes of the body. Every chakra is linked with an endocrine gland. Each is also connected to a plexus, a network of nerves. Therefore, since every chakra covers a different area of the body, some physical ailments can be directly related to a chakra that is out of balance.

Every chakra vortex is made up of smaller vortexes. Each small vortex has a different rate of vibration and a different hue. They all combine together to make a certain tone and color when they are balanced. Each mini chakra is represents one of the many aspects of that chakra. If one thing is missing in your life, it can throw off the balance of the entire chakra. Not only does each chakra need to remain balanced, all of them must be in synch for the body, mind, and spirit to function optimally.

Our Seven Chakras:

- Starting at the base of the spine, near the tailbone you will find the Root Chakra. It is red in color. This chakra is responsible for feelings of security and survival (finances, food, and shelter). This chakra regulates the testes and the ovaries.

- Moving up along the spine, located right below the belly button you will find the Sacral Chakra. It is orange in color. This chakra is responsible for pleasure, sexuality, and happiness. It regulates the pancreas.

- Moving up along the spine to the upper abdomen you will find the Solar Plexus Chakra. It is yellow in color. This chakra is responsible for self-confidence, self-empowerment, and self-respect. It regulates the adrenals.

- Moving up to the center of the chest you will find the Heart Chakra. It is green in color. This chakra is responsible for love, joy, validation, and peace. It regulates the thymus.

- Moving up to the throat you will find the Throat Chakra. It is blue in color. This chakra is responsible for the ability to communicate and express thoughts and feelings. It regulates the thyroid.

• Moving up to the center of the forehead you will find the Third Eye Chakra. It is indigo in color. This chakra is responsible for clairvoyance, decision making, and imagination. It regulates the pituitary gland.

• Moving up to the top of the head you will find the Crown Chakra. It is violet in color and is responsible for spirituality (connection to your higher self), and beauty.

It is important to keep our chakras open and functioning at the highest level possible to achieve mental clarity, spirituality to the fullest, excellent health, and emotional wellness.

The chakras are essentially energy gates of the aura. They keep our auras luminous and vivid, and when they are in balance, they will keep us healthy and happy.

How chakras radiate energy into the aura

Our life-force energy is taken into the chakra via its inward bound vortex, where it is then transported into the center or main orb of the chakra. This central area is what we tend to define as the chakra. From there, it is transported through the meridians and the central channel (the current that passes the energy through each of the chakras vertically). As life-energy flows through the body, it is picked up by each persons' DNA and passed along to the nervous and endocrine systems. At the same time, our DNA is emitting the energy all around the outside of the body, creating the aura.

Auras are our own personal energy field. The world and people around us are affected by the energy of our aura.

Auras can actually be seen as a "glowing egg" of color, glowing around the human body. The color of one's aura is determined by the strongest chakras, although, the color is a mixture of all your chakra light energy. Everyone's aura can be seen as any one of the colors in the rainbow. They appear as different hues and shades, each one having a different meaning regarding emotion, spirituality, and health.

Auras are comprised of an equal amount of layers, regardless of color. Layers differ in deepness and transparency. Most often, seven layers are seen, although it is possible for certain people to decipher nine. There is a possibility that more layers exist, but have not currently been defined.

Each chakra corresponds to a layer of the aura and are listed from 1-7, from close to the body, moving outward. The higher the number , the higher the vibration is, this causes a current of energy that moves vertically, pulsing up and out to the perimeter of the aura. The healthier the individual, and the more open the chakras, the further that the aura can extend off of the body.

7 Aura layers explained

- *Etheric Layer:* This layer ranges from a ¼ in. to 2 in. away from the edge of our physical body. The etheric layer is the medium to which our own skin is affixed. It is made up of little, delicate, threads of energy that are interwoven around the body. It is almost a copy of your skin, yet it is made of energy. Flickers of energy travel through this matrix, sparkling as they flow. Many well-practiced aura viewers can see this web of energy. Beginners may only view a muted, blurry, transparent vapor, kind of like you see coming off of the ground on an extremely hot day. May people have seen it, even if they have never tried to view an aura. It can be seen as a grey to blue fog to a novice, to sparks of blue or grey light by the well-trained eye.

The Etheric Layer is interconnected with the Root Chakra and what we experience through our five senses. This means that both physical pain and pleasure have an effect on the Etheric Body. What we eat and the way that we exercise (or lack of exercise) has an influence on it as well. The way that we feel the vibration of other's energy also takes place in the Etheric Body.

• *Emotional Layer:* Aptly named, this layer deals with our feelings and emotions. The Emotional Layer reaches out 1-3 in. from the physical body. It is a fluid layer that permeates all of the other layers. The unformulated flames of color do not resemble the shape of our physical body. The colors of the Emotional Body fluctuate in response to the emotion being felt at the time. The colors range from vivid with positive emotion, to muddy in response to negative emotion. It is possible to see every color in this layer, and it is usually the first layer of color that someone first learns to see.

Intertwined with the Sacral Chakra, the Emotional Layer is connected to how we perceive ourselves, and how those perceptions make us feel. In order to keep this layer thriving, it is important to vent and feel those emotions regardless of what they are. Do not hold them in or ignore them.

• *Mental Layer:* Like the Etheric Layer, this layer is more defined and configured. It is found 3-8 in. away from the physical body. The Mental Layer is usually seen as yellow or gold in color, and is brightest between the head and the shoulders. The radiance of the light in this layer is brightest while concentrating and focusing on a mental task. Sometimes sparks and splotches of colors are seen are seen when one creates repetitive thought patterns. These color differences are dictated by how a person is connected emotionally to their thought processes.

Our Mental Layer interacts with the Solar Plexus Chakra. It is interrelated with both left and right brain capabilities. The equal use of both sides of the brain, logical and imaginative, will keep the Mental Layer in good health. Daydreaming, lucid dreaming, the active use of the imagination, active learning, and the quest for knowledge are all things that we can do to achieve this well-being.

The Mental Layer is susceptible to serious destruction if one stays in a state of negativity or cynical thinking for too long.

- *Astral Layer:* This vaporous layer is full of color, reaching out 1-1 ½ ft. outside the body. The Astral Layer is where we create astral cords that connect us to others, whether they are positive or negative, current or previous connections.

The Astral Body is the area of the aura where we pick up on the vibrations of others. This layer is usually bathed in a pinkish color. The Astral Layer is a long term collection of how we feel about ourselves, on both an emotional and intellectual level . It is the connection linking experiences. The Astral Layer rules visualization, dreaming, and hallucinating. You are mentally aware of this part of yourself, but at the same time, you can still come into contact with other levels of reality.

The Astral Layer also allows us to project, and be in two places at the same time. The Astral Layer is connected to the Heart Chakra. This connection links us to relationships with others, and how these associations have an influence on our emotions. The way to keep this layer functioning at its best is by keeping healthy and encouraging, constructive relationships with people and the world around us.

- *Etheric Template Layer:* This layer is located around 1 ½-2 ft. outside of the body. The Etheric Template is actually a structured blueprint/ master plan of everything that is alive on the physical level.

It is a workable template of the Etheric Layer, a dark blue background with thin, light energy streaks. When something is wrong with the Etheric Layer, you can go into your Etheric Template to find out how to rebalance. This template is connected to the Throat Chakra, the place where noise is turned into matter. The Etheric Template is where divine will and the power of manifesting your will into existence are formed. Devine will is established by our inner, higher self and is the greatest longing for a direction in our existence that will serve a greater good.

By aligning our free and divine wills, we can have a healthy, vivid Etheric Template Layer. When these two wills are not lined up, this layer will still have energy lines, but they will not be as plentiful nor as bright. This will cause you to feel as if you are wandering in life without purpose. By using the power of manifestation in relation to your divine and free will, you can rebalance this layer by changing your reality and existence.

• *Celestial Layer:* While the Etheric Layer is more of a physical form of the higher self, the Celestial Layer is the emotional form of the higher self. It is located about 2-2 ¾ ft. outside of the body. The colors in the Celestial Body are iridescent and pastel, almost like a bubble or an abalone shell. In this layer we have a connection to a higher power and generate unconditional love that attaches us to other physical beings. It generates energy, much like a star or the sun, radiating outward.

The Celestial Body is associated with the Third Eye Chakra. It reflects our connections, on a spiritual level, with the universe. We can keep this layer healthy by practicing meditation, present moment awareness, and by pondering religion, spirituality, or the philosophies of reality and existence. The Celestial Layer is where we view the divine and spiritual nature within ourselves and in those around us. It also connected to each individual's awareness of the divine and how sensitive and open we are to the spiritual realm.

- *Ketheric Template Layer:* Extending 2 ½-3 ft. away from the body, this layer is where we become aware of the fact that we are one with our higher power and the universe. Its outer edge is the toughest, most durable layer.

The Ketheric Layer is oval in shape, like an egg. Comprised of thin, pulsating golden threads, it also supplies the energy that runs through the spine, powering the entire body. The higher-self fills the Ketheric Layer and this can be seen by way of a gold glow. It is the intellectual layer of the spiritual realm. Here in the Ketheric Layer we are joined with the universal mind and are able to comprehend it, as well as being able understand past lives.

The Ketheric Layer is intertwined with the Crown Chakra, and connects us to the universal mind. We can keep this layer healthy by understanding, and having insights regarding our place in the universal mind and our connection to the divine. This is achieved by having contact with higher power and having spiritual experiences. We can strengthen the Ketheric Layer by constantly seeking out divine wisdom, knowledge, and ideas.

Energy from others is taken into our aura. This can be good, if the other person has positive energy. Negative energies are what we need to be wary of as they can have a very detrimental effect on our aura.

We have quick, auric run-ins with people all of the time, but being around someone all of the time, or being in close proximity with a lot of people, negative energies are more easily absorbed. If you think that your aura has been disturbed and ingested negative energy there are purifying rituals that can rid your aura of the negativity.

Here are two examples of great visualization meditations that will cleanse your aura ~

- *The Shower:*
  Close your eyes. Visualize a shower: any kind, shape, size, even a waterfall. Decide on a shower that will allow you to feel comfortable and clean. Use your imagination and sense to experience everything: the smells, the texture under your feet, and the sound of the water.

  Step under the water and feel the water rush over your skin. Take in everything: the temperature, the smell of the water, the rush of the cleansing water over your skin. Feel the negative energy rinsing right off of your skin as the water runs down you.

  Stay in your shower until all of the negativity has washed away. Watch as the water goes down the drain or rushes away the in pool under the waterfall. The negative energy is going with it. Remain there until you are relaxed and clean.

- *The Bubble:*
  Go to a quiet, relaxing, comfortable spot. While lying down, count to twenty, slowly with your eyes closed. Imagine, in your mind's eye, a large pink bubble quite a few feet above you.

  Slowly, use all of your energy and imagination to visualize transporting all negative energy that is congesting your aura up and away from you into the bubble.

  Do this for as long as long as it takes to feel released from the negativity. Once you feel the "all clear," allow the bubble, full of the negative energy, higher and higher, up into the air until you see it disappear. Now that it is gone, you are free of that negativity.

Negative human energy is not the only kind of negative energy that can mess up your aura. The negative energy in any given location can be absorbed into the aura. Auras are prone to taking on negativity from environments like: jails, graveyards, haunted locations, various types of medical facilities, locations of frequent drug use, and many more. Try to keep your time at these kinds of places short and infrequent. Use cleansing rituals after you leave. You can keep absorption to a minimum by waving your arms around, dissipating and pushing the negative energy churning around you away. Sage (the white variety) can also be used to strengthen and stimulate your own auras positive energy. Black tourmaline is also an easy way to fend off negative energy. Some people carry it in their pocket, but a fun way to keep it with you is to have a piece of jewelry that contains it.

Knowing that the physical body is related to the auric bodies, keeping the physical health in shape will also keep our aura vivid and brilliant. Just as the circulation of the physical body is detrimental to health, so is the circulation of energy important to auric health. Eating well can help certain chakras to open up. The Heart Chakra responds to dark leafy greens. Lean proteins will help to ground the Root Chakra. The Third Eye and Crown Chakras respond well to the antioxidant properties found in dark berries and dark grapes. Not only can we eat our way to physical health, we can eat our way to auric health!

One more thing you can do to keep your aura functioning at its best is to spend time in nature. Nature is full of positive energy. Spending time out doors will help to relax the body and mind, and rejuvenate the spirit. Amp up your aura and allow nature to cleanse and heal it. Even something as simple as taking a barefoot walk in the grass or dirt is very cleansing and will ground you. Relax in the ocean, let the waves crash into you. Float down a river or wade in a stream. These natural water sources have a very cleansing quality. Nature will allow you to feel free, and give you a more positive perspective, which will in turn brighten and strengthen your aura.

THE POWER OF COLORS

Auras surround the entirety of the body, but are usually easiest to see around the head and shoulder area. We will discuss the colors and their meanings based on this area of the body.

Before we investigate the actual meanings behind certain colors, here are some added tips when reading auric color:

Most auras have 1-2 principal colors. They are known as "auric pairs" and will sometimes be the person's favorite color.

The more vivid the aura, the more aware and spiritual the person most likely is.

The more evenly that the energy is spread out in the aura more likely it is that the person is in good health.

The aura is not only comprised of dominant colors. They also contain changing flickers, sparks, or flame-like flashes that come and go. These are usually contemplations, feelings, ideas, and wants.

The color of these flashes usually falls under the definitions as follows:

- Red: An aura that is principally red usually signals a person who is very concerned with material possessions and physical appearance. Flashes of red usually indicate thoughts that are material items or something physical about the body.

- Pink (a combination of purple and red): An aura that is pink, is a combination of purple (highest frequency) and red (lowest frequency). Pink auras signal a person who has a balance of materialism and spirituality. A few people may be seen with a halo that is yellow and a huge exuding pink aura. This is a very rare dominant aura color and is usually only seen as a thought, temporarily.

- Orange: An aura that has orange as its dominant color. Orange is inspirational and fascinating. People with orange auras are inspirational and authoritative. They usually have the power to control people. When orange is a dominant color, usually a gold halo can be seen, denoting a powerful spiritual instructor. An orange flicker usually represents a thought that the person is having in regard to commanding others.

- Yellow: Someone with a yellow aura is joyful, charitable, and free. A yellow halo will only be seen on a person who is a spiritual instructor, as it signals extraordinary spiritual growth. The thickness of the halo will be one inch or less. The yellow halo is an auric pair with the violet brow chakra. Those who are working to a high level of spirituality focus attention on this chakra because they are concentrating on divine thoughts. Yellow flickers of thought signal ideas and feelings of jubilation and serenity.

- Green: People who have green auras are usually healers by nature. The more dominant and clear the green aura , the more practiced or efficient the healer. Green auras usually have a "green thumb" as well and are great at gardening. Being near a green aura will bring you tranquility and peace. When you see green flashes, this signals that the person is in a position of restoration and relaxation.

- Turquoise: Auras of this color indicate that the person is a great at multitasking, high-energy, and has great organizational skills. They like to think about many things at the same time, and have great influence over others. People with turquoise auras make great supervisors in the workplace because they go over their objectives and visions, motivating their subordinates instead of just demanding compliance. Turquoise flashes and flames indicate a thought or idea related to organization or persuading others.

- Blue: People who have dominant blue auras are tranquil, well-adjusted, and sensible. They are survivalists and can go run off to live in a cave or bunker. They would be happy to live off of the land. Blue flickers usually indicate thoughts about survival and the relaxation of the nervous system. A bright, vivid blue supersedes any auric color. It is usually seen when someone is telepathically accepting or conveying communication.

- Purple: Purple is never a dominant aura color, only as flickers of thoughts. They represent exceptionally divine thoughts.

- Darker, Smokey Colors

- Brown: Worrisome, disturbing, selfish, greedy, materialistic, thoughts that oppose divinity and spirituality.

- Grey: Morbid, discouraging, and depressing thoughts. May show unclear motives or the existence of a dark side. Mustard-like: Signals discomfort, hardship, rage, or resentment.

- White: The color white signifies problems in the aura. White color is like a racket, compared to the melodious pitch that an aura should have. White indicates discord in the person.

Before a person passes away, their aura turns white. That is why, historically, death is characterized by white, instead of black.

The understanding of auric colors will help you to understand more about your true-self, and the true nature of others. In dealing with ourselves, it helps us to see areas of improvement and where we really are on our path to enlightenment. Not only that , it can be the first step in figuring out what your strong points really are and the potential to use them to the best of your ability. Not only that, but you may see an indicator for illness, or negative energy that you could have picked up from someone else, or that you have inside of yourself. When dealing with others, our understanding of auric colors can help us to enlighten others about their true nature and possible physical and emotional health concerns. It also allows us to see past fake personalities in order to determine the kinds of people we want to allow into our lives.

CAN YOU READ AURAS?

Being able to see an aura is a very practical, insightful tool. It will help you to learn more about yourself and those around you. For most people, it takes a bit of training and practice to learn how to see an aura.

There are many different approaches and tips that will allow you to train your eyes and your consciousness to make it possible. Auras can be difficult to see at first, but once you realize that you can do it, and it clicks, you will be able to repeat the process. Naturally it is easy for kids to see auras. Babies can see them as well because they have clear, balanced chakras.

There are many ways to learn how to see auras. If you are not a "natural," do not worry, with practice you can learn how to train your eyes to see them. The techniques I have listed will aid you in figuring out how. They will also help you practice and hone your skills . Some of the methods are for use on people and others for objects. Try them all and see what works best for you. For some it may take more work, but it is possible for everyone to learn how to see auras.

Reading Other People/ White Background

- Put your subject in front of a white background with nothing on it. Make sure that there are no shadows.

- Using a colored background will make it harder. Pick a spot on the person to focus on. It will allow your peripheral vision to take over.

- You will be concentrating on one spot, and this will allow the rest of your vision to relax. Indian culture suggests that you focus on the third eye, right between the eyebrows. Stare at this spot for a minute or longer, without losing focus. This will take practice.

- Every time you find your gaze moving, refocus. After a minute, become aware of your peripheral vision.

- You must do this without taking your concentration off of your focal point. This too will take practice, and if you lose your focal point, refocus and start over.

When you do this, you should notice that the border between the body and the background has a glowing color to it. It should be a color different than the rest of the backdrop.

The longer that you focus your vision, the brighter it should become. By focusing on one spot, you are increasing your visual sensitivity to the aura. You can also allow your eyes to go out of focus, if you know how. This will allow you to pick up on other visual cues you may not have noticed.

Additional tips: Once you achieve seeing the color, have your subject shift their body from side to side. You should see their aura moving as well. Do not work on focusing for too long. Only engage in the practice for a couple of minutes at a time. Let your eyes rest in between moments of focus. If you are not seeing the aura clearly, try playing your subject's favorite music. This may invigorate their aura, allowing it to be seen more clearly.

Reading Yourself/ White Background/ Hand:

- Use a white wall or a sheet of white paper. Make sure that the lighting is natural: the sun or a candle. Do not do this at night.

- Practice in a room that is shaded from direct sunlight, if it is too bright, it will not work properly.

- Hold up a hand against the white background and let your eyes relax. Focus on the tips of the fingers or allow your eyes to become out of focus (this works best for me). Slowly but surely, you will see a clear or blue-ish glow start to form around your hand.

- Keep your gaze steady, and refocus or relax again as necessary. Eventually the brightness will turn into a color.

- Decide exactly what colors you are seeing.

Additional tips: Sometimes you will see an "after image" or a negative looking effect. Do not base your auric color on this. You will be able to tell if it is a negative image if you look away from your subject matter and wherever you look you will see the same image inversely. Just like when you stare at a bright light for a long period of time and see it no matter where you look for a minute or so afterward.

Also, do not worry if you start to see the color and it disappears quickly. Blinking your eyes and loss of focus is common. Afterwards, it is helpful and fun to take a white piece of paper and draw an outline of your body. Using colored pencils, pastels, whatever you like , sketch out the colors you see. You can keep them on hand, for your own personal reference, or just to show others.

Do not get discouraged if you do not see anything right away. You have to relax, practice, and train your eyes . Try these exercises when you are relaxed and in a place free of distraction. If sunlight is not working for you, use a dark room only illuminated with candlelight.

Reading Yourself/ Mirror

- Have large mirror about four feet in front of you.

- Try to make sure that the background behind you is white.

- You should see to it that there are as few shadows as possible.

- The lighting should be constant and soft.

- Follow the same instructions above (as when you used your hand).

Do this for 10 15 minutes every day. This will help you to train your eyes to see auras.

Additional tips: Once you are able to see your inner-aura, the bluish, white glow, you can try your hand at seeing color. As in the previous exercise, place yourself in front of the mirror. Focus on seeing that same inner aura again, but now, try to concentrate on the border of that glow.

With practice, the glow will grow wider. You should be slowly able to see color start to border the edge, and it may be hazy, or dim at first. This is how you be able to see the color of the middle aura. It will take time, but step by step you should become more comfortable with it.

From here you can move on to seeing the shape of the aura. You will need all the materials in the exercises above, but this time a full length mirror would be helpful. Find the border, your white glow, and relax your vision to see the other colors. Start with your head, and when you lose focus, simply bring it back. It is a practice of refocusing your attention.

As you get more skilled, you can train your eyes to see the aura in front of the body, not only around it. Once you are focused, follow the aura from one side of the body to another. Across the top of the head is a good place to try: move from one shoulder, over the head, to the other shoulder. After you master that, try looking at the front of you, even down your torso, groin and legs.

Reading Yourself/ Fingers

- Place your hands together, press your pointer tips together. Pull them apart just a bit.

- Concentrate your gaze in between them. You are trying to focus on waves of energy passing between them, kind of like heat waves on a warm asphalt parking lot.

- Relax your vision every so often and let them go out of focus intermittently.

Another option, using your digits, stretch one of your arms out directly in front of you. Put your hand into a fist, thumb facing up. Move the thumb to eye-level. Now, concentrate you gaze on the tip. Hold your focus, without blinking for as long as possible. If performed correctly, you should be able to make out whips of energy, right there at the tip.

How to see the aura of a tree

Trees are large and produce an aura that can be huge, strong, and clearly visible. Try to do it around dawn or in the evening. Pick a tree that is tall, broad, and stands alone. Stand approximately 20 feet away from it. Focus on the tree's outline. It should be a hazy, green/ gay color. You will see this outline between the sky and the tree most often faintly at first, then once you have caught a glimpse of it, let your eyes go out of focus a bit or squint slightly. Practice for as long as you need to. You can try other trees as well.

How to see the aura of a plant

Find a plant that is still. Potted plants work well for this exercise. Find a spot to focus you attention on, either near the top or the base. Allow your eyes to relax and go out of focus. This can also be accomplished by focusing slightly beyond the plant. Slowly, the white aura of the plant should begin to appear. You may not see the same colors you would when reading a person's aura, but it is still a useful practice. It will help to train your eyes to see other auras.

Practicing Tips and Tricks

1. Practice your sensing skills. Be aware of how you feel around others. What "vibe" are they giving you? Are they pulling from your energy or adding to it? While paying attention to their energy, focus on your breathing. Note what your physical senses are telling you, how they are making your mind and body feel. Practice picturing the color this person makes you feel. You may not always be correct, but it is a great way to start sensing aura. Visualization and sensation go hand in hand.

2. Practice using your peripheral vision. This is an ability that most people have, but because we do not always use it in everyday life, it must be strengthened . It is also an area of sight that has not incurred as much damage as the rest of the eye. You can practice for a minute or so at a time by focusing sight on one spot. It will heighten your sensitivity, and you will notice a big difference in your focus in the far corners of your vision.

3. Practice with colors. Find a white solid background, like a wall, and make sure the lighting is mellow, no direct glare. Wrap a book in a bright primary colored paper and stand it up on a table, facing you, white wall in the background. Place yourself a few feet away. Take a few cleansing breaths with your eyes closed, open them looking directly at your subject. Practice on focusing on the border of it, even a little bit past

it. You should start to see a thin, glowing border. Keep your focus and you should notice it turning a greenish-yellow. This can be done with many objects and colors. It will help you train your eyes to see color that our everyday vision does not always pick up. When you lose focus during a practice such as this, do not worry, you are not doing it wrong. Stay relaxed and refocused, the more you do it the better your eyes will be at balancing themselves this way.

4. Quick fixes: honing your aura reading skills can be done all the time. There are little things you can do anywhere. Gauge the aura of a customer or co-worker. Focus on them and you may notice a difference in it as they become angry, frustrated, comfortable, or pleased. When at the beach, look at the border of the water on the horizon. The top of a crest of a crashing wave is also electrifying. Nature holds many aura-frying sights, which if we remain still and focused, can blow our minds. A simple man-made key can be a wonder. Hold it in your hand for fifteen minutes. Seal your energy into it. Put it down, and visualize your energy in the key, you should actually be able to see your emotion fixed onto it.

Do not lose faith if you are not picking it up right away. As we move through life some people become desensitized to the process. In order to strengthen and train that ability we have to practice! You can develop the skill to see auras, just do not give up. 15-20 minutes of practice goes a long way. Try to practice every day . The ability to sense energy takes time. As you make little steps, you will gain more confidence in your abilities. Confidence plays a huge part in the ability to see auras.

BALANCING AURAS FOR OUR PHYSICAL AND EMOTIONAL HEALTH

It is just as important for us to keep up our energy body as it is for us to keep up our physical body, yet many people neglect it. Our life energy not only affects our physical and mental health (and vice-versa), it also brings things into our life, and repels others. Keeping our auras bright and healthy allows us to stay in great emotional and physical shape as well. Sadly, especially in this day and age, our life-energy body can become neglected. Now that you are aware of this, you have the power to fix it easily.

The balancing and cleansing process will not only help you to feel energized, think clearly, have control over your emotions, it will help you to deflect negative energy and pass positive energy to others. Not only is it possible to pick up negative energies from others, we can also produce it in ourselves. Negative thoughts about ourselves and past experiences create bad energy. The wrong diet, lack of exercise, or use of drugs (prescriptions included) and alcohol can also taint the aura with negative energy. This causes an imbalance or blockage in the flow of our life energy.

We know what happens when our energy is blocked or unbalanced. The aura will suffer as well as our physical being. You can become sick, feel lethargic, nervous, disheartened, or emotionally and mentally unstable. It is possible to balance and clear our flow of energy, and achieve wellness by cleansing the aura.

There are many different methods of aura cleansing available. Most are super practical and easy to use! Many of them are also beneficial to your physical health, so why not try them? Did you know that even drinking 12 glasses of spring or purified water a day will not only help the physical body detox but it also will help to purify the aura? I find that using all methods in combination works well. You will enjoy engaging in these aura cleansing techniques and finding out which ones work best for you.

Bathe in sea salt.

Yes, something as simple as taking a bath in dissolved sea salt is very cleansing for your aura. We have to wash our spiritual body just like we was our physical body. This type of bath takes away negative energy while strengthening the aura. Sea salt builds a type of barrier that protects against negative energy. Sea salt is very grounding and will pull out undesirable spiritual energy from the skin. Water is purifying by nature and will cleanse our positive energy. After a sea salt bath you will be left with a protected and cleansed aura.

Different people conduct this bathing ritual in various ways. The most important things to include are a previously bathed body, sea salt, and an undisturbed period of time. 15-30 minutes is recommended. Your favorite essential oils can be added, you can burn incense, play calming music, or a guided meditation.

- Fill your bathtub with warm water and dissolve a cup or two of sea salt into it. I relax my entire body, a section at a time, bottom to top.

- Next, I visualize all of my stress, worry, self-doubt, and negative feelings brought on by others being sucked out of my body through the skin.

- Try to make sure all of your body is submerged at one point or another.

- When you are done, get out of the bath knowing you are clean and free of any negativity.

I also find that a dip in the ocean works in the same way. It is cleansing and freeing. Although you should be wary of polluted areas, as this may counteract the effect.

Light

Light visualization is easy to do. I prefer to use this method out in the sunlight, to double the effect, but it can be done indoors as well.

- Lie down in a comfortable place.

- Take a few cleansing breaths and close your eyes.

- When you are completely relaxed, visualize a white light above you. I use the sunlight that permeates my eyelids, but either will do.

- Feel the light come into your body, filling every inch of it. As it engulfs the body, imagine it taking the place of negative energy.

- Imagine the light cleansing and repairing the entirety of your body. Relish in the moment.

- After you have done this for a while, visualize extending the light outside of your body. See it pushing out all negative energy. Feel all of your negative energy leaving your body and moving far away from you.

The light has now restored your energy and replaced all negativity.

Deep Breathing

Deep breathing is very cleansing for your aura. This one is simple by nature, but is sometimes tricky to get the hang of.

- The more you practice, the easier it will become. Once a day, find a quiet spot where you will be undisturbed. At first do this exercise in 5-10 minute increments and then work up to half hour sessions.

- You should sit comfortably and close your eyes. Start by inhaling for four seconds. Exhale for four seconds. Each time you inhale feel the breath penetrate deep down into your stomach.

- Concentrate on your breathing as you to this. You are focusing attention only on the inhale and the exhale of your breath. Every time you get distracted, simply redirect your attention to your breath. Continue this process until you are fully relaxed.

- After a few minutes, each time you inhale imagine that you are inhaling a white, glowing, flow of energy. As the breath enters your body, imagine that you are filled with a glowing white light.

- Feel the light restoring your body and your energy.

- Upon exhaling, see your breath coming out as dark negative energy.

- Experience the feeling of relief as you push out negative energy. Each time your lungs empty, experience a peace knowing that your energy is balanced.

Use a sage stick for smudging away negative energy.

It is an ancient cleansing process that sounds "hocus-pocus-y," but really works.

- Simply purchase one at a new age or health food store.

- Light one end of the stick.

- When you see a flame, blow it out and it should begin to smolder.

- Swirl stick around yourself as the smoke encircles you.

- The smoke will rid you of bad energy.

Crystals also work well to cleanse the aura and protect it.

There is much to learn about the science behind crystals, how to use them in healing, and how they protect the aura. Here are a few basic ways you can easily use crystals for cleansing. When in doubt, or for more complicated crystal usage consult a professional.

- One good thing that crystals are great for is to protect a cleansed aura from negative energy. Black Tourmaline can be carried with you. Rose Quartz is good as well because it substitutes negative energy for positive energy.

- Labradorite keeps people from sucking away at your positive energy. It will protect your aura from being leeched off of by others.

- Amethyst, Bloodstone, Citrine, and Quartz are all great cleansing stones.

- You can use these stones by carrying them on your person, waving them around you through your aura, wearing them on a piece of jewelry, or putting one next to your bed.

- You can also meditate with a crystal.

Here is an easy way for a beginner to practice an aura cleanse. Find a quiet place and lie down. Practice some deep breathing mediation for a few minutes with your crystal placed on your third eye chakra. Now visualize a white glow coming from the crystal. Allow the light to course through your body, and then around it. Let the light purify your aura, as it encircles your body in a cleansing glow. Do this until you feel refreshed and clean.

Essential oils are fabulous aura cleansers and are very easy to use. You can have them mixed professionally, or choose a single oil to use on your own. If you have company coming over or grumpy kids in the house, diffusing essential oils will help set the mood and adjust attitudes! Cleansing and creating a more enjoyable atmosphere for everyone.

Common cleansing oils are: lime, juniper, cinnamon, cypress, and lemon.

- Make your own aura misting cleanser by using a clean spray bottle, filling it with a cup of spring water, and adding a couple of drops of the essential oil of your choice. Mix it will and spray yourself!

- You can add a few drops of essential oils to a cleansing bath. Easier still, using your finger, put a few drops at your neck and the inside of your wrists and ankles. Inhale the aroma left on your fingers with slow deep breaths while you imagine your aura brightening as you inhale, and negativity exiting with your exhale.

Those are many practical, everyday ways you can easily cleanse your aura. How can you tell if your methods work? You will feel cleansed, at ease, of sound mind, and positive... back to yourself.

You don't have to do them every day, but consistency is key. Find what works best for you. If you do not feel like these methods are working for you. I encourage you to see someone who specializes in energy healing. As a cautionary reminder ~ not everyone will have your best interest at heart. Be mindful and follow your intuition when choosing someone.

Living a peaceful and balanced life

Life is a journey that we are all on. In order to make the most of it, it's important to live a healthy and balanced lifestyle. This is not only important for our own personal journey , happiness, spiritual health, and physical wellbeing, it is detrimental to those around us.

It's very important to be mindful of the atmosphere you are creating for yourself and exposing others to. It not only sets the mood but tells other's how to behave and how to treat you!

The energy of the universe is alive in all of us, and we are alive in it. Everyone plays a part in each other's existence. If you want to be a beneficial element, radiating healthy, vibrant energy, it is important to learn how to understand and feel our own energy in order to see how it has an effect on our own health, circumstances, and relationships.

When you consider where we came from, non-physical pure energy of the universe, and where we are today, physical energy, and you understand that we are both forms of energy its really amazing! The journey we traveled in both non-physical and physical combined to create who we are. When we were born we didn't have a veil limiting us from ourselves. It was created by the beliefs we learned growing up and as we continue to expand, it is those beliefs we shed allowing us to connect on a deeper level to the non-physical side of ourselves. For it is in this non-physical side that we will find the answers we seek and the balance we desire.

When I look around at people I can see inside of them. I can see where they came from, the choices they have made along the way, and where they are going in the future. Every day we have choices placed in our path and each choice leads to another path. Neither choice is wrong, and both come with lessons to learn on the way before we receive the outcome we desire. As you look at the choices before you, you will notice one choice will always feel like you are fighting the current and the other will feel like it's going with the natural flow... For this day and all the days before you, may you always pick the one that flows...

Free yourself!

Many Blessings with Love and Light,

    Cindy